The Sheldon Short Guide to
Diabetes

Mark Greener spent a decade in biomedical research before joining *MIMS Magazine* for GPs in 1989. Since then, he has written on health and biology for magazines worldwide for patients, healthcare professionals and scientists. He is a member of the Royal Society of Biology and is the author of 21 other books, including *The Heart Attack Survival Guide* (2012) and *The Holistic Health Handbook* (2013), both published by Sheldon Press. Mark lives with his wife, three children and two cats in a Cambridgeshire village.

Christine Craggs-Hinton, mother of three, followed a career in the civil service until, in 1991, she developed fibromyalgia, a chronic pain condition. Christine took up writing for therapeutic reasons and produced more than a dozen books for Sheldon Press, including *Living with Fibromyalgia*, *The Chronic Fatigue Healing Diet*, *Coping Successfully with Psoriasis* and *How to Manage Chronic Fatigue*. She moved to the Canary Islands, where she became the resident agony aunt for a local newspaper and also took up fiction writing. Christine died in 2013.

GW00535891

Sheldon Short Guides

A list of titles in the Overcoming Common Problems series is also available from Sheldon Press, 36 Causton Street, London SW1P 4ST and on our website at www.sheldonpress.co.uk

THE SHELDON SHORT GUIDE TO
DIABETES

Mark Greener and
Christine Craggs-Hinton

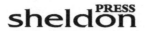

First published in Great Britain in 2016

Sheldon Press
36 Causton Street
London SW1P 4ST
www.sheldonpress.co.uk

The author and publisher have made every effort to
ensure that the external website and email addresses
included in this book are correct and up to date at the
time of going to press. The author and publisher are
not responsible for the content, quality or continuing
accessibility of the sites.

British Library Cataloguing-in-Publication Data
A catalogue record for this book is available from the
British Library

ISBN 978–1–84709–382–0
eBook ISBN 978–1–84709–383–7

Typeset by Fakenham Prepress Solutions, Fakenham,
Norfolk NR21 8NN
First printed in Great Britain by Ashford Colour Press
Subsequently digitally reprinted in Great Britain

eBook by Fakenham Prepress Solutions, Fakenham,
Norfolk NR21 8NN

Produced on paper from sustainable forests

To Yasmin, Rory, Ophelia and Rose, with love

Contents

A note to the reader

This is not a medical book and is not intended to replace advice from your doctor. Consult your pharmacist, diabetes nurse or doctor if you believe you have any of the symptoms described, and if you think you might need medical help.

A note on references

We used numerous medical and scientific papers to write the book that this Sheldon Short is based on: *The Diabetes Healing Diet*. Unfortunately, there isn't space to include references in this short summary. You can find these in *The Diabetes Healing Diet*, which discusses the topics in detail.

Introduction

People living with diabetes have dangerously high blood sugar levels that poison their cells. Over several years, the raised levels of sugar can cause debilitating, distressing and disabling complications, such as pain, ulcers, amputations, heart disease and blindness. However, combining drugs, diet and other lifestyle measures could avoid most of these complications and may even reverse the early, gradual increase in blood glucose levels that ends in the most common form of diabetes. Even if you're taking medicines, a healthy, balanced diet increases your chances of avoiding diabetes-related damage, disability and death. This short book outlines the lifestyle changes – and diet in particular – that can help you tackle diabetes and live a fulfilled, active, satisfying life.

This book discusses general principles. It does not replace advice from your diabetes nurse, doctor or GP. They offer support tailored to your problems and circumstances. Rather, the book aims to support their expert advice. If you have any questions, speak to your diabetes team. Diabetes UK (<www.diabetes.org.uk>) is an invaluable source of advice and support. Never adjust or stop any medicine without speaking to your doctor or diabetes nurse.

In addition, everyone with diabetes should take part in 'structured education' courses, which cover lifestyle, medications and monitoring blood glucose. For instance, DAFNE (Dose Adjustment For Normal Eating) and DESMOND (Diabetes Education and Self-Management for Ongoing and Newly Diagnosed

Diabetes) help people with types 1 and 2 diabetes, respectively. Speak to your GP or diabetes team about local courses.

1

The pancreas – controlling glucose levels

Cells are, essentially, biological factories. They use a sugar called glucose as fuel. We extract glucose from carbohydrates (such as sugars and starch) we eat and drink.

Carbohydrates are long chains of sugars. Starch, for example, consists of long chains of glucose. Sucrose (table sugar) contains glucose joined to another sugar called fructose. Digestion breaks carbohydrates into single sugars, carried around your body in your blood.

Insulin stimulates cells to take glucose from the blood. Without insulin, most cells cannot use glucose. So, blood glucose levels rise in people who do not produce enough insulin. Levels also rise if insulin does not work properly when it reaches the cells (insulin resistance).

High levels of glucose can cause serious damage. So, people with diabetes urinate more to flush the excess sugar out of the body – and their urine tastes sweet. In 1674, Thomas Willis, a leading English doctor, used the sweet taste to distinguish diabetes from other diseases that caused frequent urination, such as infections or bladder stones. Willis coined the term 'diabetes mellitus' – the latter term from the Greek word for honey or sweet.

To understand why a healthy, balanced diet helps people with diabetes, we need to look at how the body normally controls blood sugar levels. We'll begin with the pancreas.

The pancreas

The pancreas, which is about 15 cm (6 inches) long, lies behind your stomach (Figure 1). The rounded 'head' is next to the first part of your bowel after your stomach (duodenum; Figure 2). Your pancreas has two vital roles, producing:

- pancreatic juice, a cocktail of chemicals that helps you digest food, and
- several important hormones, including insulin.

Pancreatic juice

Food travels from your mouth, down the food pipe (oesophagus) and into your stomach. Acid in the stomach sterilizes, and starts digesting, food. Food then flows into the duodenum (Figure 1).

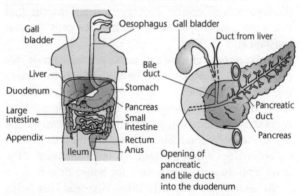

Figure 1 The digestive system

Figure 2 The pancreas

Specialized cells in the pancreas (acinar cells) pump pancreatic juice into small ducts. These feed into a larger channel running the length of the organ – the pancreatic duct (Figure 2). Meanwhile, the liver and gall bladder (a small pouch under the liver) release a greenish-yellow fluid called bile, which helps digest fats. The gall bladder stores bile. Bile flows along ducts from the liver and gall bladder. These join to form the common bile duct and enter the head of the pancreas. The common bile duct and pancreatic duct converge, then join the duodenum.

Islands in a pancreatic sea

When the nineteenth-century German medical student Paul Langerhans examined the pancreas under a microscope, he saw small, pale 'islands' in a 'sea' of acinar cells. We now know that these Islets of Langerhans produce hormones that control blood sugar levels.

Each of the million or so islets contains three major types of cell:

- Beta cells produce insulin. The term 'insulin' comes from the Latin for island: *insula*.
- Alpha cells produce glucagon, which essentially has the opposite actions to insulin.
- Delta cells secrete somatostatin. This, in turn, controls the release of other hormones, including glucagon. (Hormones are a type of chemical messenger, carrying signals around the body.)

Pancreatic islets produce several minor hormones. We won't consider somatostatin or these other hormones further.

Insulin

Insulin is so important that the protein differs little between mammals. That's why injections of insulin from cows and pigs can treat diabetes in a human. Even dung beetles produce insulin. So why is insulin so important?

We obtain most of the glucose we need from starchy carbohydrates (such as rice, pasta, potatoes, bread) and sugars in, for example, fruit and sweet foods. Digestion breaks starch and sugars into glucose.

Blood glucose levels shoot up within a few minutes of swallowing a sugary drink. Converting starchy carbohydrates into sugars takes longer, which helps smooth out peaks and troughs in blood sugar. This steady supply helps everyone stop snacking between meals. A steady supply also helps people with diabetes avoid potentially dangerous declines in blood sugar (hypoglycaemia).

As your cells need glucose all day, you have various stores, including in your liver and kidneys. After a meal, blood glucose levels rise rapidly, triggering insulin release. In response, glucose release from the liver declines by almost 80 per cent. The sight and taste of food also triggers insulin release, which helps your body prepare for the surge in glucose. Several other parts of the diet, such as amino acids (building blocks of protein) and fats, stimulate insulin release.

Insulin levels rise in parallel with the increase in blood glucose, which returns to pre-meal concentrations after around three hours. So, insulin secretion drops. About half the insulin released by the pancreas follows the spike in blood glucose levels after a meal. You slowly release the rest during the day. Doctors can use several types of therapeutic insulin to mimic this natural pattern.

Insulin's actions

Insulin stimulates cells to take up glucose from the blood. When insulin levels fall, cells switch to alternative energy sources, such as fat.

Some organs – including the brain – don't store glucose and cannot use alternative sources (see below). These organs need a constant supply of glucose. Indeed, your brain uses around a quarter of all your glucose. So, insulin stimulates the liver to stick glucose into a long chain called glycogen. Muscles store glycogen for future use – a bit like a biological battery. Broken back into glucose, typical glycogen stores would keep an average woman going for a day.

The liver's storage capacity is limited. But glucose is too valuable to waste. So, liver cells convert additional glucose into fatty acids, which other tissues use as fuel when there's not enough glucose. This conserves glucose for organs (such as the brain) that cannot use fatty acids. Meanwhile, fat cells use glucose to make another chemical called glycerol. Glycerol joins with fatty acids forming fats called triglycerides – another energy store. Unfortunately, high levels of triglycerides increase the risk of heart disease and pancreatitis (inflamed pancreas).

Insulin also stimulates cells to take up amino acids. When insulin levels are low and we have depleted other energy stores, cells break down protein in our muscle. This releases amino acids. The liver converts some amino acids into glucose (gluconeogenesis).

Glucagon: insulin's partner

Glucagon has the opposite effect to insulin: it increases blood glucose levels. So, when blood glucose levels fall, glucagon secretion increases, which:

- triggers liver cells to break down glycogen stores, releasing glucose;
- activates gluconeogenesis;
- stimulates the breakdown of triglycerides into fatty acids.

Exercise triggers glucagon release, at least in part because working out burns up glucose. The interplay between insulin and glucagon tightly controls blood glucose levels.

2

Types of diabetes and their symptoms

Essentially, diabetes arises when insulin no longer tightly controls levels of blood glucose. Diabetes has at least 50 possible causes. However, type 1 diabetes mellitus (T1DM), which usually starts during childhood, and T2DM, which typically emerges in overweight, middle-aged people, are the most common.

Type 1 diabetes mellitus

Our immune system targets harmful bacteria, viruses and parasites. To limit 'collateral' damage to healthy tissues, proteins called antibodies 'stick' to the invaders and trigger the immune reactions. Occasionally, however, the immune system produces antibodies against healthy tissues (autoantibodies, a process called autoimmunity), which, depending on the target, can cause rheumatoid arthritis, multiple sclerosis or T1DM.

T1DM accounts for about one in ten cases of diabetes in adults. In T1DM, environmental factors seem to interact with a genetic predisposition to trigger the immune system to produce autoantibodies that destroy beta cells. So, people with T1DM need regular insulin injections.

The environmental triggers are something of a mystery, although infections probably contribute. For example, children born to women who contract rubella (German measles) during pregnancy seem particularly prone to developing T1DM. Some studies suggest a link between T1DM and introducing cow's milk relatively early in an infant's diet. So, a short duration of breast-feeding may increase the risk.

Type 2 diabetes mellitus

T2DM accounts for most cases of diabetes. Excess weight causes about nine in every ten cases of T2DM, by triggering three main changes. Their relative importance differs from person to person and doctors don't yet know which comes first:

- low insulin production
- insulin resistance
- abnormalities in a group of hormones called incretins (see below).

Most people with T2DM show all three to a greater or lesser extent. All three are progressive. So, T2DM usually gets gradually worse, often despite medicines.

Low insulin production

In early T2DM, patients do not secrete enough insulin to cope with high glucose levels after a meal (postprandial level). The low insulin levels also mean that the liver doesn't reduce glucose production properly, which contributes to high postprandial blood sugar levels. As T2DM progresses, beta cells become less effective. So, insulin production declines. In turn, blood glucose levels rise, even between meals. By the time he or she is diagnosed, a person with T2DM has typically lost 50–70 per cent of beta cell function.

Insulin resistance

As T2DM progresses, muscle, liver, fat and other cells gradually respond less and less well to insulin. These 'insulin-resistant' cells take up less glucose from the blood. In early T2DM, the pancreas produces more insulin to overcome the resistance. This increased production, together with poisoning by high glucose levels, damages the pancreas. Eventually, damaged beta cells cannot produce enough insulin to overcome the resistance.

Incretin abnormalities

In T2DM, a group of hormones in the gut – incretins – stop working properly. Glucose in food normally triggers incretin release. In turn, incretins increase insulin secretion. This allows the body to prepare for the surge in glucose after a meal. Patients with T2DM typically lose a quarter of their incretin function before they are diagnosed.

Humans produce two main incretins, called:

- GIP – glucose-dependent insulinotropic peptide; also known as gastric inhibitory peptide.
- GLP-1 – glucagon-like peptide-1.

Drugs targeting incretins are a mainstay of treatment for T2DM.

Prediabetes

T2DM usually develops over many years. So, there's a grey area between normal blood glucose levels and diabetes. This stage – called 'prediabetes' – doesn't usually cause symptoms but can still damage your body. About one person in ten with IGT (see box) or early diabetes shows damage to the delicate, light-sensitive layer at the back of their eyes (retinopathy). The progression to full-blown diabetes isn't inevitable. A healthy diet and lifestyle can reverse prediabetes.

Diagnosing prediabetes

Doctors use two diagnostic tests to detect prediabetes:

- Impaired fasting glucose (IFG; also called impaired fasting glycaemia) measures your blood sugar level after you've not eaten ('fasted') overnight. IFG can miss 20–30 per cent of cases of T2DM.
- Impaired glucose tolerance (IGT) measures blood glucose after you have fasted for eight to ten hours. The doctor takes another blood sample two hours after you swallow a drink containing a known amount of glucose. IGT assesses your risk of serious problems more accurately than IFG.

Other types of diabetes

There are several less common types of diabetes.

Gestational diabetes

Gestational (during pregnancy) diabetes may arise because the pancreas does not produce enough insulin to meet the increased demands of having a baby. Overweight and obese women are particularly likely to develop gestational diabetes. Pregnancy may also uncover existing diabetes.

Gestational diabetes usually resolves after the baby's birth. However, women with gestational diabetes are about three times more likely to develop T2DM. Poorly controlled diabetes can also harm unborn babies. So, ensure good control of blood glucose before and during pregnancy. Make sure you take sufficient folic acid (folate) before and during pregnancy: women with diabetes need higher doses of this essential vitamin.

Maturity-onset diabetes of the young

Maturity-onset diabetes of the young (MODY) is a genetic disease that knocks out beta cells' ability to sense changes in blood glucose levels. Many people with MODY are probably misdiagnosed with T1DM or T2DM. Lifestyle changes, such as a healthier diet and increased physical activity, can treat many cases of MODY.

Pancreatitis

Chronic (long-term) inflammation of the pancreas can destroy insulin-producing cells as well as being painful and life threatening. Indeed, 40–60 per cent of people with chronic pancreatitis have diabetes. Pancreatitis can arise from high levels of fat (especially triglycerides) in the blood and excessive alcohol consumption. But doctors can't find a cause for many cases of pancreatitis.

Secondary diabetes

Occasionally, drugs and surgery trigger 'secondary' diabetes. Not surprisingly, secondary diabetes emerges immediately after surgeons remove a diseased pancreas. Certain medicines – such as steroids and thiazide diuretics ('water tablets') – can trigger diabetes.

Diabetes insipidus

Diabetes insipidus arises when, for example, infection, injury or drugs, such as lithium used to treat bipolar disorder (manic depression), undermine the body's ability to regulate water levels. Affected people produce very large amounts of dilute, watery urine.

Symptoms

Some diabetes symptoms emerge as the body tries to deal with the high levels of glucose. So, people with diabetes mellitus urinate more – especially at night – and tend to feel thirsty. Other symptoms – such as feeling tired and weak – emerge because cells can't use glucose to generate energy.

Less commonly, the rise in insulin levels in early T2DM and overweight people can cause acanthosis nigricans – dark, thick velvety patches around the groin, neck, armpits and other body folds. The high insulin levels increase skin cells' activity.

Often, however, a serious complication is the first sign of diabetes. The first sign of T1DM may be ketoacidosis – a potentially dangerous rise in blood sugar levels. In people with T2DM, a heart attack, eye damage or a slow-healing wound may be the first indication. And see your doctor if you have any of these symptoms:

- more frequent urination than usual, especially at night;
- being very thirsty or drinking excessively;
- feeling hungry;
- extreme tiredness and constant fatigue;
- unexplained and sudden weight loss;

- genital itching or regular episodes of thrush;
- cuts, sores and wounds that heal slowly;
- skin infections (especially recurrent);
- blurred vision;
- tingling and numbness in the hands and feet.

3

Risk factors for diabetes

We can't do anything about some risk factors for diabetes – such as our genes. But many risk factors are within our control. This chapter looks at the most important.

Obesity and being overweight

Broadly, we have two types of fat. Subcutaneous fat just below the skin conserves body heat. Abdominal (visceral) fat continuously pumps out chemicals that carry messages around the body.

High levels of some of these chemicals are one reason why being overweight – even just carrying a few extra pounds – increases the risk of developing diabetes. On the other hand, if you can lose about 5–7 per cent of your weight – that's about 4.5–6.8 kg for someone who weighs 90 kg – you may be able to postpone T2DM.

Ethnicity and waist size

T2DM usually occurs in obese and overweight people over 40 years of age. However, T2DM appears earlier and is more common in certain ethnic groups. So, the cut-off for dangerous abdominal obesity is lower for people of some ethnic backgrounds (Table 1).

Table 1 Waist sizes linked to increased risk of health problems

| | Waist size | |
	Health at risk	Health at high risk
Men	Over 94 cm (37 inches)	Over 102 cm (40 inches)
Women	Over 80 cm (32 inches)	Over 88 cm (35 inches)
South Asian men	–	Over 90 cm (36 inches)
South Asian women	–	Over 80 cm (32 inches)

Source: Adapted from the British Heart Foundation

Risk factors cluster

You're more likely to develop T2DM if you're overweight. You're also more likely to develop dangerously raised blood pressure (hypertension) if you're overweight. And if you have diabetes, hypertension increases your risk of developing heart disease more than if you just had raised blood pressure alone. In other words, risk factors cluster.

The landmark INTERHEART study, published in *The Lancet*, compared about 15,000 patients from 52 countries who experienced their first heart attack with roughly the same number who had never had a heart attack. Researchers identified nine factors that accounted for 90 per cent of the risk of the first heart attack in men and 94 per cent among women (Table 2 overleaf). INTERHEART also found that:

- smoking just one to five cigarettes a day increased

heart attack risk by 38 per cent compared with life-long non-smokers;

- heart attack risk roughly doubled in those smoking six to ten cigarettes a day and increased almost four-fold in those smoking between 16 and 20 cigarettes a day;
- the risk of a heart attack rose to just over ninefold in people smoking at least 41 cigarettes a day;
- diabetes and hypertension each roughly doubled the risk of the first heart attack.

On the other hand,

- eating fruits and vegetables daily (30 per cent reduction), regular exercise (14 per cent reduction) and

Table 2 Factors linked to the risk of suffering a first heart attack in the INTERHEART study

Risk factor	Increase in heart attack risk
Hypertension alone	2 times
Diabetes alone	2 times
Smoking alone	3 times
Abnormal lipid profile (dyslipidaemia)	3 times
Hypertension, diabetes, smoking	13 times
Hypertension, diabetes, smoking, dyslipidaemia	42 times
Hypertension, diabetes, smoking, dyslipidaemia, obesity	69 times
Hypertension, diabetes, smoking, dyslipidaemia, psychosocial factors	183 times
Hypertension, diabetes, smoking, dyslipidaemia, psychosocial factors, obesity	334 times

Source: Adapted from Yusuf S, et al. Lancet 2004;364: 937–52.

regular alcohol consumption (9 per cent reduction) protected against the first heart attack. As we'll see later, a healthy diet and exercise also help control diabetes.

INTERHEART showed that clusters of risk factors dramatically increase heart attack risk:

- People with diabetes who smoke and have hypertension are 13 times more likely to experience a heart attack than those without any of the nine risk factors.
- Those with diabetes and four other risk factors (harmful fat levels, obesity, smoking and hypertension) are almost 69 times more likely to have a heart attack.
- If you have enduring psychosocial problems (such as stress and depression) in addition to diabetes and the other four risk factors, you are about 334 times more likely to have a heart attack than those without any of the nine risk factors.

Metabolic syndrome

People who are prediabetic and those with diabetes often show a cluster of risk factors called metabolic syndrome. Definitions vary, but if you have at least three of the following, a doctor may diagnose metabolic syndrome:

- diabetes or IFG, or you are taking a drug for diabetes;
- a waistline of at least 94 cm in European men and at least 80 cm in European women (cut-offs differ for certain ethnic groups);
- abnormal lipids (dyslipidaemia), such as low levels of high-density lipoprotein (HDL) in your blood,

or you're taking a medicine (such as a fibrate or niacin – ask your GP or pharmacist if you're not sure) to boost levels of this 'healthy' fat;

- high levels of triglycerides, or you're taking medicines to cut levels of this harmful fat;
- hypertension, or you're taking a medicine to reduce your blood pressure.

If you have one risk factor ask your GP or nurse to check for others. Doctors and patients should treat each component in addition to a healthy lifestyle.

Healthy and lethal cholesterol

Despite its bad press, cholesterol is an essential part of the membranes around every cell and the insulation surrounding many nerves that ensures signals travel properly. Cholesterol is also the backbone of several hormones.

To get around the body, cholesterol attaches to 'transporters' called lipoproteins. One of these, low density lipoprotein (LDL), carries cholesterol from the liver to the tissues. LDL accumulates in artery walls, forming fatty deposits called plaques that cause most heart attacks and many strokes. Another lipoprotein, HDL, carries cholesterol away from the arteries and back to the liver for excretion, cutting the risk. It's easy to remember: LDL is 'lethal'; HDL is 'healthy'.

Alcohol and diabetes

Alcohol can trigger pancreatitis and helps pile on the pounds. So, not surprisingly, excessive alcohol consumption increases T2DM risk. However, moderate consumption may reduce T2DM risk by heightening cells' sensitivity to insulin, lowering circulating levels of insulin or both.

Alcohol poses other risks for people with diabetes. For example:

- If you're using insulin or certain antidiabetic tablets, you need to remain within limits agreed with your diabetes team to avoid hypoglycaemia.
- Alcohol can increase triglyceride levels. Many people with diabetes have high levels of these fats, which are linked to heart disease, in their blood.
- Alcohol can exacerbate the pain from neuropathy caused by diabetes and further damage nerves.
- Regularly drinking more than three to four units of alcohol a day can exacerbate retinopathy.

Polycystic ovary syndrome

Women with polycystic ovary syndrome (PCOS) develop numerous cysts around the edge of their ovaries that contain underdeveloped eggs. All women have some such cysts. But most women with PCOS have many more, which often cannot release their egg.

Although the cause of PCOS remains enigmatic, hormones seem to be important. All women, for example, produce small amounts of some 'male' hormones, such as testosterone. But women with PCOS produce markedly higher levels or the hormones are particularly active. Furthermore, many people with PCOS produce excessive levels of insulin, for example because they are overweight, which seem to contribute to the increased production and activity of male hormones.

PCOS symptoms usually emerge in the late teens or early 20s. Some women experience menstrual problems, such as no, irregular or light periods, or find that they can't conceive. Other women gain weight or develop excessive body hair, oily skin and acne, and hair loss. Later in life, obesity, hormone imbalances and insulin resistance characteristic of PCOS increase the risk of hypertension, abnormal levels of LDL and HDL, and diabetes.

4

Complications of poorly controlled diabetes

Raised levels of blood glucose can 'poison' cells. Over several years, this can cause distressing and disabling diabetic complications such as:

- microvascular complications including neuropathy (nerve damage), nephropathy (kidney disease) and retinopathy (eye damage);
- macrovascular complications including heart disease, stroke and peripheral vascular disease – a blockage in the blood vessels supplying the limbs;
- other complications including a higher risk of infections, impotence, problems during pregnancy and, in children, impaired growth and development.

Taking medications, measuring and controlling blood glucose and a healthy lifestyle can reduce the risk of complications.

Checking blood glucose levels

Raised blood glucose levels – a potentially serious condition called hyperglycaemia – rarely cause symptoms, but can still damage your health. So, your diabetes team may suggest that you check your levels regularly using a self-testing kit. This is essential if you're using insulin or some other treatments for T2DM.

Your team may also suggest that you monitor blood glucose levels, for example to determine if you need antidiabetic tablets or insulin, to ensure you're taking the right dose and to help plan and assess lifestyle changes.

Some blood glucose monitoring devices store readings. But keeping a diary allows you to note your activities at the time you took the measurement, what you ate and how you felt. Over time, you'll see how changes in your lifestyle influence your blood glucose levels. Your diabetes team will help you decide when to test and your target blood glucose level.

Other checks

In addition, see your doctor at least once a year to check:

- your feet and legs, to see if your feet are becoming numb (a sign of nerve damage);
- your blood pressure: hypertension increases the risk of heart attacks, strokes and kidney disease;
- your cholesterol (LDL, HDL and total) and triglyceride concentrations;
- your kidneys: persistently high blood glucose levels can damage your kidneys leading to protein 'leaking' into your urine (microalbuminuria or albuminuria).

See your optician – at least once a year but more often if you have diabetic eye disease – and your dentist regularly. Make sure they know you have diabetes.

Urine testing

Measuring sugar levels in urine is less painful than drawing blood. But it's also less accurate and may miss potentially important changes in blood glucose levels. The body starts flushing excess glucose out of the body at blood levels higher than those that can cause complications: even a trace of glucose in your urine means that your blood levels are too high. Furthermore, some people with normal blood glucose levels excrete sugar in their urine, either during pregnancy or because they have a genetic condition called renal glycosuria. So, it's best to measure blood glucose levels.

HbA_{1c}: a different perspective

A blood glucose measurement tells you the level at that time. It doesn't take account of the peaks and troughs over the days, weeks and months. So, your doctor or diabetes nurse should measure your HbA_{1c} (glycosylated haemoglobin) level at least once a year.

HbA_{1c} measures glucose carried by red blood cells. Glucose 'sticks' to the haemoglobin that carries oxygen (biologists call this glycosylation). So, measuring HbA_{1c} indicates your blood glucose levels for the previous two or three months – the lifespan of haemoglobin. You'll agree an HbA_{1c} target that is right for you with the diabetes team. You need both HbA_{1c} and regular blood glucose measurements to provide an accurate picture of your diabetes control and the impact of changes to your drugs, lifestyle and diet.

Hypoglycaemia

In hypoglycaemia (sometimes spelt hypoglycemia) blood sugar falls to very low levels and there isn't enough glucose to fuel your activities. Early hypoglycaemia symptoms include:

- hunger
- sweating
- shaking and trembling
- weakness
- rapid heartbeat, fast pulse, palpitations
- numb and tingling in and around the lips
- headache
- blurred vision
- dizziness
- looking pale.

If you don't correct the low blood levels, you may develop intermediate symptoms, such as:

- difficulties with thinking and concentrating
- double vision
- poor coordination
- fatigue
- confusion
- irritability, nervousness, anxiety.

Persistently low levels can cause unconsciousness and seizures. The pattern of hypo-related symptoms differs between people and can change over time in the same person. Several factors increase the risk:

- poor coordination between the dose of insulin and eating or activity;
- some antidiabetic tablets;
- delaying or missing a meal or snack;

- not eating enough carbohydrate;
- taking part in unplanned or especially strenuous activity;
- drinking too much alcohol, especially on an empty stomach;
- lack of food overnight.

Keeping a diary of blood glucose readings, when hypos occur and the symptoms can help you identify how to improve control. For instance, changing the type of insulin may help prevent hypos during the night.

Treating hypoglycaemia

Severe hypoglycaemia can end in unconsciousness, coma or a fit. So, if you have any of the symptoms or your blood glucose measurements suggest you're at risk (ask your doctor or nurse if you are not sure), immediately consume between 10 and 20 g of a rapidly acting carbohydrate, such as:

- a glass of Lucozade, a non-diet soft drink or fruit juice
- at least three glucose tablets (carry these with you)
- five jelly babies or other sweets
- two tablespoons (20 g) of dried fruit, honey or syrup.

Test your blood glucose levels again after 15 minutes. If your blood glucose is still too low, consume another 10–20 g of rapidly acting carbohydrate.

Once you're back in the target range, eat some long-acting carbohydrates to stop your blood glucose from falling again. For example, if your next meal isn't due in 15 minutes after you're back in the target range, eat one of the following:

- half a sandwich

- some fruit
- a small bowl of cereal – carry some cereal bars or fruit with you
- biscuits and milk.

Hyperglycaemia and ketoacidosis

Hyperglycaemia can arise if blood levels rise too high, causing, for example:

- increased thirst
- frequent urination
- lethargy and lack of energy
- headaches
- stomach pain.

Numerous factors can trigger hyperglycaemia, including:

- missing a dose of insulin
- using insufficient insulin
- eating more carbohydrate than usual
- over-treating hypoglycaemia
- stress
- infections.

You need to get rid of the excess glucose from your blood. So, drink large amounts of sugar-free fluids, and you may need another dose of insulin. You may need to test for ketoacidosis. If you experience hypoglycaemia or hyperglycaemia frequently, speak to your diabetes team to help you improve control.

Ketoacidosis

When cells cannot use glucose, you begin to 'burn' fat. This creates toxic by-products called ketones (sometimes called ketone bodies), which the body excretes in urine. So, people who produce large amounts of ketones often become increasingly thirsty. If you produce more ketones than your body can handle, you may develop the symptoms of ketoacidosis, such as:

- frequent urination
- excessive thirst
- increased appetite
- blurred vision
- abdominal pain or discomfort
- heavy, deep (called Kussmaul) breathing
- nausea and vomiting
- dehydration
- acetone on the breath – may smell similar to pear drops or nail polish (nail polish contains acetone, which smells similar to pear drops)
- confusion and lethargy.

Your diabetes care team will advise when you need to check your ketone levels, usually by dipping a testing strip into a urine sample or using an electronic device. The combination of high levels of ketones and blood glucose can produce a potentially fatal coma. So, rapid treatment is essential.

If your ketone levels are high (especially if your blood glucose levels are high) call your doctor or diabetes nurse immediately or go to your nearest A&E department. If your ketone levels are high and you feel very unwell – if you feel drowsy, breathless or nauseous, or you are vomiting – ask another person to take you to A&E or ring for an ambulance.

Diabetes and infections

People with diabetes are especially vulnerable to infections. High blood sugar levels can undermine the immune system. Bacteria and fungi – such as the yeast that causes thrush – use sugars to fuel their growth. And your body uses a lot of energy to tackle illness and fight infections. So, blood glucose levels rise and some cells respond less well to insulin when you're ill – even if you lose your appetite or are off your food.

Ask your GP or diabetes nurse for advice while you feel under the weather. Don't stop taking your insulin and test your blood glucose level as advised by your GP or nurse. Make sure that a close family member or friend knows how to check your blood glucose and adjust your medication in case you feel too sick. Wear a medical alert bracelet to let people know you have diabetes – if you're unconscious, for example. If you don't have one, ask your GP or diabetes nurse.

Diabetes and heart disease

People with diabetes are between two and four times more likely to have a stroke, develop angina or suffer a heart attack than people without diabetes. Allowing for other factors, deaths following heart attacks are a third higher among people with diabetes. So, why are people with diabetes at such high risk?

The development of plaques

Even if we don't have diabetes, fatty material starts collecting inside our arteries from early childhood, sometimes even in the womb. Gradually, these deposits develop into atherosclerotic plaques, which cause many heart attacks and strokes. As a plaque enlarges, the bore down the middle of the blood vessel narrows. Depending on the site of the plaque, the reduced blood supply can cause health problems, including chest pain (angina), kidney damage and impotence.

Plaques form around damage to the vessel's normally smooth inner lining caused by, for example:

- diabetes
- excessive levels of fat in the blood
- dangerously high blood pressure
- changes linked to age
- nicotine and other toxins from smoking.

The damage triggers the sequence leading to an atherosclerotic plaque (Figure 3).

The damage allows fats and certain white blood cells to enter the vessel wall. Some white blood cells engorge with fat. Meanwhile, chemicals released by white blood cells:

- promote inflammation around the damage;
- increase the amount of muscle and collagen (a type

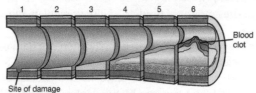

Site of damage
1 Damage to the inner lining of the blood vessel
2 Fatty streak forms at site of damage
3 Numbers of white blood cells increase, inflammation and small pools of fat appear
4 Large core of fat develops, and amounts of muscle and collagen increase
5 Fibrous cap covers a fat-rich core, while calcium deposits harden the plaque
6 Plaque ruptures, triggering a blood clot

Figure 3 Development of an atherosclerotic plaque

of protein that enhances strength and flexibility) in the blood vessel wall;

- recruit even more white blood cells into the damaged area.

These changes help patch the damaged vessel wall. But it's a short-term fix. As fat continues to pour from the blood into the plaque, muscle cells form a cap covering a core of cells, fat and debris from dead cells. Capillaries grow into the plaque. But these are fragile, so blood leaks into, and further swells, the plaque. Calcium deposits gradually harden the plaque.

A balanced diet and a healthy lifestyle dramatically reduce the risk of heart attacks, strokes and peripheral arterial disease. Your doctor may prescribe one or more drugs to, for example, lower blood pressure (which can rupture plaques) or reduce levels of dangerous fats in your blood. The British Heart Foundation (<www.bhf.org.uk>) offers more information.

Chronic kidney disease

Kidneys filter blood, keeping useful salts and water and expelling waste, including excess glucose. As they control the amount of fluid, the kidneys regulate blood pressure.

High levels of glucose and hypertension can damage the vessels inside the kidneys that filter blood. So, waste and superfluous fluid stays in the circulation. This pushes blood pressure higher. Unless treated, this cycle of damage may end in a transplant or dialysis. Indeed, diabetes and hypertension are leading causes of chronic kidney disease (nephropathy). On the other hand, controlling blood pressure and glucose levels protects against kidney damage.

Most of us have more kidney function than we need. So, mild chronic kidney disease doesn't cause symptoms. But as the damage progresses you may develop:

- tiredness
- swollen ankles, feet or hands caused by water retention
- shortness of breath
- itchy skin
- nausea
- problems having or keeping an erection.

People with kidney disease excrete protein in their urine (albuminuria or proteinuria). Doctors and nurses can test for this by dipping a special strip into your urine. Small increases in albumin (the most common protein in blood) in the urine (microalbuminuria) can identify early kidney disease long before symptoms emerge. Certain drugs may slow the progression of kidney disease. So, check whether you've been tested recently.

Impotence and erectile dysfunction

Between 35 and 90 per cent of men with diabetes experience erectile dysfunction – they can't gain or keep an erection hard enough for intercourse. Numerous factors may contribute:

- certain conditions linked to diabetes, including raised levels of cholesterol and other fats, hypertension and obesity;
- some diabetic complications, such as neuropathy, nephropathy and peripheral vascular disease;

- several medications (including some drugs used to treat hypertension);
- smoking and excessive alcohol intake.

So, swallow any embarrassment and speak to your doctor, who can offer Viagra (sildenafil) and other treatments for erectile dysfunction.

Up to a quarter of women with diabetes experience sexual dysfunction, including pain during intercourse and changes in desire, arousal or orgasm. Urinary tract infections and vaginal thrush – which are common among women with diabetes – can contribute. Doctors, nurses and counsellors can often resolve these problems.

Nerve damage

Up to half of people with diabetes develop nerve damage (neuropathy). This can hinder transmission of nerve signals from the brain and spinal cord to muscles, skin and other organs, and vice versa. The damage can cause severe pain, potentially debilitating complications and 'autonomic' symptoms, which include constipation, diarrhoea, impotence, dry skin and poor awareness of hypoglycaemia.

Good control of blood sugar may prevent, partially reverse and slow the progression of painful diabetic neuropathy. Doctors can suggest a range of pain-killers (analgesics) and other treatments for painful neuropathy.

Foot ulcers and amputations

Diabetes can damage nerves that carry messages from your feet to your brain. So, you may not realize when you tread on something sharp, develop a blister due to tight footwear or the bath is too hot. This means you are more likely to suffer minor injuries and you're less likely to protect these small wounds by not walking on them. You might not realize that a stone in your shoe is burrowing into your sole. This damage can quickly worsen and develop into ulcers – especially as the skin may not heal as well in people with diabetes.

Severe foot ulcers can lead to amputations. A blocked artery supplying a limb can lead to the cells dying, causing gangrene. Again, this can end in amputation. Indeed, amputations are 10 to 30 times more common in people with diabetes than among the general population. According to Diabetes UK, there are 135 diabetes-related amputations in England a week – that's one every 75 minutes.

Many people with T2DM mistakenly regard poor blood circulation as the main cause of lower limb numbness, discomfort and amputation. So, they try to improve the blood supply to their feet by regularly walking barefoot or wearing open-toed sandals or footwear a size too large 'to give the toes space to move'. Ironically, this could increase the chance of injury.

So, see a chiropodist, podiatrist or foot protection team regularly. Between appointments, inspect your feet each day, and see your doctor if you find cuts and splits between your toes or discolouration to your feet and toes.

Eye disease

Patients with diabetes are 10 to 20 times more likely to go blind than people with normal blood glucose levels. Indeed, diabetes is the main cause of blindness among people of working age in the UK. Poorly controlled diabetes can damage nerves in the hands. So, people left blind from diabetes may not be able to read Braille. People with diabetes are also twice as likely to develop cataracts (cloudiness in the lens) or glaucoma (increased pressure exerted by the fluid inside the eye, which damages the retina).

High blood levels of glucose can damage the tiny blood vessels supplying the retina, the light-sensitive layer at the back of the eye. As a result, blood, fluid and fat leak into the retina. New blood vessels form as the body tries to bypass the damage. But these immature vessels are fragile and may burst. Blood flows into the eye causing sudden loss of vision. Over time, scar tissue can push the retina from the underlying tissue. These changes occur even before your vision alters, so get your eyes checked each year.

Depression and anxiety

Diabetic complications can be distressing and debilitating. If you experience a potentially fatal complication, such as a heart attack or stroke, you may live in fear for your life. Tightly controlling blood glucose can impose a considerable mental toll, especially as you juggle other commitments or feel guilty about the time you spend managing your disease or the impact on your family. Not surprisingly, depression and anxiety are common in people with diabetes.

Don't underestimate depression or anxiety

Depression is more than feeling 'down in the dumps'. It's profound, debilitating mental and physical lethargy, a pervasive sense of worthlessness and intense, deep, unshakeable sadness. Anxiety is more than feeling a little wound up, worried or stressed out. It's intense, overwhelming, sometimes debilitating, fear – even terror. If you've never experienced 'clinical' depression or anxiety, it's difficult to appreciate how devastating the conditions are.

Sometimes changing your diabetes medications or lifestyle may improve your blood glucose levels and, in turn, alleviate this cause of anxiety or depression. In general, putting yourself in control of your problems is one of the best ways to beat anxiety and depression. In contrast, feeling that your diabetes (or another problem) controls you commonly causes anxiety, depression and stress. Unfortunately, people living with depression or anxiety may be less motivated to stick to lifestyle changes and diabetes treatments, which increases the risk of complications.

Your doctor may suggest antidepressants or drugs to alleviate anxiety (anxiolytics). Don't dismiss drugs. They don't cure the underlying problem. But antidepressants or anxiolytics may offer you a window of opportunity to improve control of your diabetes and deal with any other issues you face. It's often difficult to plan the best way to overhaul your lifestyle to help control your diabetes or tackle other problems when you're living with depression or anxiety.

Many people find that talking to a counsellor helps. Ask your GP or contact the British Association for Counselling and Psychotherapy (<www.bacp.co.uk>).

Cognitive behavioural therapy

Counsellors and psychotherapists may use cognitive behavioural therapy (CBT) to help you identify feelings, thoughts, behaviours and beliefs associated with diabetes. CBT then helps identify which mental strategies are unhelpful and unrealistic, and replaces these with more appropriate responses. CBT can help you face issues that you have avoided and try out new ways of behaving and reacting, which bolsters your psychological defences, overcomes practical issues and helps improve your control of diabetes.

Stress

Even if you don't suffer full-blown anxiety or depression, living with diabetes can leave you stressed out. So, your body pumps out hormones and other chemicals to get you ready to fight or run away. Blood glucose levels rise to provide extra energy. This helped when we faced a sabre-toothed cat or a rival tribe: the threat was relatively short-lived and we burnt excess glucose off. However, dealing with an over-demanding boss, financial problems and a chronic disease rarely offer the chance to relax. So, blood glucose levels remain high, which can undermine the control of your diabetes. Exercise and eating patterns can also suffer.

So, be particularly careful about monitoring your blood glucose levels when you're stressed. Try using relaxation CDs, learning to meditate, massage, hypnotherapy (<www.bamh.org.uk>) or the many books now available to tackle stress.

5

Treating diabetes

People with T1DM need regular insulin injections. Some people control T2DM with diet and lifestyle alone. But 80–90 per cent of people with T2DM need one or more injectable and oral medicines, which may include insulin. And new treatments for diabetes regularly reach the market. Each has benefits and disadvantages. So, you should be able to find the right drug, or combination, that controls your blood sugar and reduces the risk of complications. There's not space here to look at each drug. So, speak to your diabetes nurse, GP or contact Diabetes UK.

Modern medicines for diabetes are generally effective and relatively safe. But drugs aren't a replacement for lifestyle changes. You need to do both. This chapter looks at some lifestyle changes that reduce your risk of developing T2DM, improve control of blood glucose levels and help prevent diabetic complications. We'll look at diet in the next chapter.

Losing weight

Being overweight is the main risk factor for T2DM. (Ironically, some drugs for diabetes cause weight gain.) Losing weight, especially abdominal fat, improves cells' sensitivity to insulin, reduces levels of unhealthy fats and lowers blood pressure.

If you have a medical condition (including diabetes), speak to your doctor before you start dieting. A dietician – speak to your diabetes team or contact the British Dietetic Association (<www.bda.uk.com/>) – can help find the best weight loss programme for you.

How to lose weight – and keep the pounds off

Losing weight is not easy – whatever the latest fad diets would have you believe. Millions of years of evolution drive us to consume food to help us survive during times of famine. And you can't stop eating as you can quit smoking. But the following may help:

- Set yourself a realistic, specific goal by a particular time. Don't say that you want to lose weight: rather, resolve to lose, say, 2 stone (13 kg). Eating 500–1,000 fewer calories each day can reduce body weight by between 0.5 and 1.0 kg each week. Use an on-line body mass index (BMI) calculator (see <www.nhs.uk/Tools/Pages/Healthyweight calculator.aspx>) or ask your doctor or nurse to set your target.
- Stick to your exercise programme.
- Keep a food diary. Record everything you eat and drink for a couple of weeks. It's easy to pile on calories: extra biscuits, glasses of wine or full-fat lattes soon add up.
- Think about how you tried to lose weight in the past. What techniques and diets worked? Which failed to make a difference or were you unable to stick to?
- Tightly control your blood glucose. Snacking can prevent hypoglycaemia but can encourage weight gain.

- Choose foods that keep you feeling full for longer.
  For example, eat complex carbohydrates that slowly
  release their glucose rather than simple sugars.
- Don't let a slip-up derail your diet. Try to identify
  the triggers. A particular occasion? Do you comfort
  eat? More frequent hypos? Once you know why you
  slipped you can stop the problem.

If you need additional help, you could ask your
doctor or diabetes care team about local weight
loss support groups. Diabetes UK offers advice and
support about weight management. GPs, diabetes
nurses and pharmacists can suggest medicines to
kick-start weight loss, though you'll still need to diet.

Exercise

Glucose fuels your body's activities. The more you
exercise the more fuel you need. So, exercise lowers
blood glucose levels and aids weight loss. Exercise also
increases mobility, strength and stamina, and helps
protect your bones, heart and cardiovascular system.
Finally, exercise strengthens your immune system,
combats stress and promotes sleep.

Start slowly and increase the amount that you
exercise as and when you feel able. Aim at being mod-
erately active for at least 30 minutes on at least five
days a week, and ideally every day. It doesn't have to
be in one go. You can exercise for 15 minutes twice a
day, for instance.

Exercise until you are breathing harder than usual,
but not so hard that you can't hold a conversation.
You should feel that your heart is beating faster than
usual and you've begun to sweat. If you experience
chest pain, stop exercising and see your doctor. You

may need to monitor your blood sugar level especially carefully when you increase your exercise. Ask your diabetes team if you're uncertain what to do.

Make exercise part of everyday life

Find an exercise that suits you and fits into your lifestyle. If you're not a natural water baby or the pool is some distance from home or work, you may be more likely to quit exercise based on swimming. The following are relatively easy to fit into a busy life:

- *Walking* for about 30 minutes four or five times a week. An electric treadmill gives you the freedom to walk whenever you wish, whatever the weather. If treadmill walking seems monotonous and artificial, try reading, watching television or listening to music or podcasts while you exercise.
- *Swimming* once or twice a week works the major muscles and encourages deeper breathing. Gradually build up to an hour-long session.
- *Cycling* using an exercise bike or outdoors.
- *Participation sports*, apart from keeping fit, help you meet new people. Ask your sports centre, adult education centre or library about local clubs. You'll find something that suits you.

Look for opportunities in your everyday life to become more active, such as:

- Walk to the local shops instead of taking the car.
- Ride a bike to work instead of travelling by car.
- Park further away, say a 15-minute walk, from your place of work.
- If you take the bus, get off one or two stops early and walk the rest of the way.

- Use the stairs instead of the lift.
- Clean the house regularly.
- Instead of using a carwash, clean the car by hand.
- Take up gardening.

Quit smoking

Everyone knows that smoking increases the risk of heart disease, strokes and cancer. Smoking, however, can make matters worse for people with diabetes. For example:

- Diabetic kidney damage is more common and, once nephropathy develops, worsens more quickly in smokers than non-smokers.
- Nerve damage is more common and worsens more quickly in people with diabetes who smoke compared with non-smokers.
- As we have seen, people with diabetes are especially likely to develop heart disease and stroke. But smoking further increases the risk of heart disease and stroke in people with diabetes.
- Smoking can make breathing difficult, so your ability to exercise declines.

Tips to help you quit

Quitting reduces your likelihood of developing most smoking-related diseases. However, fewer than one smoker in every 30 manages to quit annually. More than half of these relapse within a year. So, try the following:

- Set a date when you will stop completely.
- Plan ahead: keep a diary of situations that tempt you to light up, such as coffee, meals, pubs or work breaks. Find an alternative.

- Find something to take your mind off smoking. If you smoke when you get home in the evening, distract yourself with television, a hobby or exercise. The craving usually only lasts a couple of minutes.
- Smoking is expensive. Note how much you save and spend at least some of it on yourself.
- Learn to deal with stress and hunger pangs. Don't reach for the sweet packet. Monitor your blood glucose especially carefully if quitting smoking changes your eating habits.
- Nicotine replacement therapy increases quit rates by between 50 and 100 per cent. Nicotine patches reduce withdrawal symptoms but begin working relatively slowly. Nicotine chewing gum, lozenges, inhalers and nasal spray act more quickly. Talk to your pharmacist or GP to find the right combination for you.
- Many people have quit using e-cigarettes. These don't contain the cancer-causing chemicals in tobacco. But as e-cigarettes deliver nicotine they remain addictive, and we still don't know if there are any long-term health risks. So, again, e-cigarettes can take you a large step towards kicking the habit, but don't stop there.
- If you still find quitting tough, doctors can prescribe other treatments. But you'll still need to be committed to quitting.
- Some people find hypnotherapy helps them quit. Contact the British Association of Medical Hypnosis (<www.bamh.org.uk/>).

Nicotine is incredibly addictive and many people don't quit first time. But if you relapse, try not to become too dispirited. Regard it as a temporary setback, set another quit date and try again. Identify why you relapsed. Were you stressed out? If so, why? Was smoking linked to a particular time, place or event? Once you know why you slipped you can develop strategies to stop the problem in the future.

6

Diet and diabetes – the first steps

Overhauling your diet can seem daunting. But many people find that it takes only a month or so of eating (or not eating) a food for it to become a habit. You'll soon become accustomed to unsweetened drinks and less salt, for example. The improvements in your health and appearance make it easier to keep following a healthy diet.

Keep a food diary

Recording everything you eat and drink, when, and, if you take them, your blood glucose levels, helps identify problems with your current diet – such as where extra calories creep in – and aspects of your everyday life that affect control. If you have prediabetes or are controlling T2DM with lifestyle alone, the food diary helps identify changes that could make a difference.

You may think you know how much junk food, vegetables, sugar and alcohol you consume. But guesses are often wrong. One study, for example, found that, on average, we underestimate calories by one-fifth. According to Alcohol Concern (<www.alcoholconcern.org.uk>), average drinkers underestimate consumption by the equivalent of a bottle of wine each week.

You'll need a notebook or computer or smartphone app. Some people begin by recording snacks, drinks and extra sugar. This eases them into note-making. When you have kept a full food diary for a couple of weeks your dietary pattern and the effect on blood glucose levels should emerge. As you improve your diet, the food diary shows just how far you've come in taking control of your diabetes.

Controlling carbs

Broadly, two main types of carbohydrate supply energy:

- complex starchy carbohydrates, including rice, chapattis, yam, noodles, cereals, pasta, potatoes and bread;
- simple sugars including caster, granulated and other table sugars, and fruit sugar (fructose). Dairy foods, pies, pastries, biscuits and cakes contain simple sugars.

Some food labels refer to monosaccharides and disaccharides – saccharide is the chemical term for sugar. The mono- and di- refer to the number of sugars – mono- is one, di- is two. So glucose is a monosaccharide. Sucrose is a disaccharide.

Sucrose (table sugar) contains glucose joined to fructose. Carbohydrates are long chains of sugars. Starch consists of long chains of glucose, for example. Digestion breaks carbohydrates into single sugars, of which glucose is the most important.

Blood glucose levels rise after we eat carbohydrates. The size of the peak and how long glucose remains raised depends on the type of carbohydrate and, to a lesser extent, other components of our diet. For example, glucose levels rise within a few minutes of swallowing a sugar-laden drink. Converting whole-wheat pasta into glucose takes longer. So, complex carbohydrates have longer-lasting effect on blood glucose levels than simple sugars.

Glycaemic index and glycaemic load

Glycaemic index (GI) ranks foods' effect on blood glucose. Weight for weight, foods that contain large amounts of slowly absorbed carbohydrate produce a steady rise in blood glucose with a relatively low peak – a bit like a gentle hill. These foods are lower GI. Foods containing high levels of simple sugars produce a more rapid rise and a higher peak – more like a mountain – and are higher GI.

Scientists test the effect of 50 g of a food on blood glucose levels over two to three hours. They compare the rise to that produced by 50 g of glucose or white bread, which scientists define as a GI of 100. So, they can rank GI for different foods. For example, 50 g of bread does not have the same effect on blood glucose as 50 g of fruit. Both differ from 50 g of pasta. Some breads that include whole grains have a lower GI than the same weight of wholemeal (where the whole grain is ground up) or white bread.

Low GI carbohydrates help maintain relatively con-stant blood glucose levels:

- A low GI meal helps you avoid hypos, ironing out peaks and troughs in glucose.
- Slow-acting carbohydrates reduce the marked peaks in blood glucose following a meal, which may help prevent T2DM.
- Low GI foods help you lose, or stay at a healthy, weight. The slow release of glucose means you feel

Table 3 Examples of low, medium and high GI foods

Glycaemic index		Food
Low	Less than 55	Apples, oranges, pears, peaches
		Beans and lentils
		Pasta made from durum wheat, noodles
		Sweet potato (peeled and boiled)
		Sweetcorn
		Porridge, All-Bran, Special K, Sultana Bran
		Custard
		Wholegrain breads
		Some raw fruits
Medium	55–70	Honey, jam
		Shredded Wheat, Weetabix
		Ice cream
		New potatoes (peeled and boiled)
		White basmati rice (cooked)
		Pitta bread
		Couscous
High	70–100	Glucose (e.g. tablets)
		White and wholemeal bread
		Brown and white rice (cooked)
		Cornflakes
		Baked and mashed potatoes
		White bread
		Biscuits
		Sugary drinks

fuller for longer. So, you're less likely to snack between meals.

- Low GI diets may reduce heart disease risk and raise levels of healthy HDL-cholesterol.

Table 3 shows some examples of various foods' GI. Obviously, this isn't comprehensive. So read the label, buy books that include the GI values or use lists on the internet.

Limitations of the GI

The GI helps you make healthy food choices. But it has limitations:

- Whether you compare a food with glucose or with white bread can influence GI. One brand of toasted bread was high GI compared with white bread and medium compared with glucose.
- Low GI isn't necessarily healthy. Ice cream is often medium GI. Chocolate is low or medium GI. Both are high in saturated fat. Potato crisps are medium GI. A baked potato is high GI, but is healthier than fat- and salt-laden crisps.
- Eating sufficient fibre can be difficult if you're eating a low-carbohydrate diet. A high-fibre diet helps prevent constipation, aids weight loss, reduces cholesterol and protects against colon (bowel) cancer.
- Be careful using international tables. The composition of the same brand may differ between countries.
- The GI of some foods seems to be increasing, partly as manufacturers try to make food preparation and cooking easier and quicker. The GI of porridge oats can depend on the refining, for instance.

- We don't eat single foods. We eat bread and butter, 'meat and two veg' or pasta and sauce. Fat and protein can hinder carbohydrate absorption. Liberal dollops of sugar-rich jam means you digest low GI granary bread more quickly. Mashed potato is high GI – adding cheese reduces the GI but increases the fat. A baked potato is high GI – adding tuna, baked beans or cheese makes the meal low GI. So, think about the meal overall.

Glycaemic load

GI is based on 50 g of the food. However, a slice of bread may weigh 30 g, while a typical portion of frozen peas may be 80 g. Obviously, portion size influences the amount of carbohydrate and, therefore, the effect on blood sugar. Glycaemic load (GL) also considers portion size. Foods are split into three GL groups:

- high: GL of 20 or more
- medium: GL of 11 to 19
- low: GL of 10 or less.

Some sugar-packed drinks, certain bagels and cakes have GL over 20. Almost all low GL foods have a low GI. In between, it's more complex. A breakfast cereal could have a GI of 72. But the 30 g serving gives a GL of 18. So, it's high GI, medium GL.

GL can seem confusing – although books and internet lists can help. As GL uses the same principle as GI, many of the same criticisms apply. So, some health professionals may feel both are too complex and variable for everyday use. They tend to emphasize a healthy, balanced – rather than a low-carbohydrate – diet. You need to think about the calories, fibre, vitamins and minerals, even if GI or GL helps. A dietician can give you individual advice: contact your diabetes team or the British Dietetic Association.

Carbohydrate counting

You can use food labels to count carbohydrates and adjust your dose of insulin. Basing insulin doses on carbohydrate counting may allow more flexible diets, while enhancing blood glucose control.

Basically, look at the total carbohydrate in 100 g of the food. Don't use the 'of which sugars' value. Check the portion or serving size, which can be considerably less than you eat. That gives the carb count. Check whether the amount is cooked or not. You can use carb counts to keep your intake constant and to estimate how many grams of carbohydrate one unit of insulin will cover. Your diabetes team can let you know more about carbohydrate counting.

Non-sugar sweeteners

Sugar can creep into your diet in many ways including:

- sucrose (white table sugar)
- brown sugar (such as muscovado and Demerara)
- icing sugar
- raw sugar, in the form of granulated crystals
- glucose – sometimes called dextrose
- honey, which contains glucose, maltose and sucrose.

Many sugar-free and low-calorie foods and drinks replace sugar with a 'polyol' sweetener, such as sorbitol, maltitol, xylitol, isomalt or mannitol. Polyols have fewer calories than sucrose and the body doesn't absorb all the carbohydrate. So, polyols have less effect on blood glucose levels than sucrose. As a result, people may need less insulin when they eat polyol sweeteners. However, excessive consumption of polyol sweeteners can produce diarrhoea and flatulence, especially in young children.

Celebrations

Just because you're diabetic doesn't mean you have to miss out on birthday cakes, parties and Christmas celebrations. If you generally eat a healthy diet, occasional celebrations won't do any long-term harm, but watch your blood glucose levels closely and you may need to adjust your dose of insulin. Many celebratory foods are loaded with calories, fat and sugar. Meals often tend to be larger than usual. And it's easy to become distracted – and eat more than you planned.

Make sure the meal includes plenty of fruit, vegetables and starchy carbohydrates. That's a good idea for everyone, not just those with diabetes. You could try offering vegetable crudités, olives and dried fruit as an alternative to high-fat snacks and chocolate. Finally, get off the sofa – even walking around the January sales helps.

7

Diet and diabetes –
beyond carbs

Changes in carbohydrate consumption cause fluc-
tuating blood glucose levels. But don't become too
hung up on carbohydrates. You could miss important nutrients. A healthy, balanced diet maintains
and improves everyone's health, not just those with
diabetes.

Alcohol

Everyone should watch how much alcohol they drink.
But people with diabetes should be particularly careful.
Alcohol lowers blood glucose levels, often for several
hours. While people with diabetes with stable blood
glucose levels can enjoy social drinking, they must be
on guard against hypos. If you're at risk of hypos your
diabetes team will often agree a limit on your drinking
with you. This may differ from the safe drinking levels
outlined in the box.

Some hypo symptoms (such as staggering, passing
out and confusion) can resemble drunkenness. If
your breath smells of alcohol, doctors may think that
you're drunk and miss your hypo. So, always carry
diabetes ID (such as a bracelet, card or necklace) with

> ### *A UK unit of alcohol*
>
> You should discuss the alcohol consumption that's right for you with your doctor. One unit of alcohol contains 8 g alcohol. So:
>
> - Half a pint of normal strength beer, lager or cider equals one unit.
> - One small (100 ml) glass of wine equals one unit.
> - A large (175 ml) glass of wine equals two units.
> - A single (25 ml) measure of spirits equals one unit.
> - One 275 ml bottle of alcopop (5.5 per cent/ volume) equals 1.5 units.
>
> An American 'drink' contains 14 g of alcohol or just less than two UK units.

you – speak to your diabetes team or GP if you don't have any.

If you feel hung over, check your blood glucose to ensure that the headache, nausea, shaking and sweats aren't caused by a hypo. Try your best to eat some breakfast. But if you can't face food (or you are vomiting), drink as much fluid as you can, including some sugary drinks. And don't stop taking your insulin or other antidiabetic medication.

Carbohydrate in alcoholic drink

In brewing and winemaking, yeasts convert sugar in grain or grapes to alcohol. However, alcoholic drinks contain widely different amounts of carbohydrate, so read the label:

- Dry wines and spirits contain little or no carbohydrate.

- Beer, lager and cider contain moderate amounts of carbohydrate.
- Alcopops, sweet sherry, sweet wines and port contain large amounts. Low-alcohol beers may be higher in sugar.
- Low-sugar brands convert more of the sugar to alcohol.

Drinking safely

If you want to drink:

- Stay within safe drinking levels: ask your diabetes team or GP.
- Have drink-free days each week.
- Don't drink on an empty stomach. Have a meal before you go out or within half an hour of your first drink. If you can't, eat carbohydrate-containing snacks such as a sandwich, nuts or crisps throughout the time you're drinking.
- Make sure family or friends know what to do if you have a hypo. Drinking may make you less aware of a hypo's warning signs.
- Alternate alcoholic beverages and either water or sugar-free soft drinks. This slows alcohol consumption and helps avoid dehydration.
- Use diet drinks, soda or water as a mixer with spirits. A shandy made from beer or lager and lemonade, for instance, is high in sugar.
- You're at risk of a hypo for several hours after you stop drinking. So, eat some food – such as cereals or toast – before going to bed to help avoid nocturnal hypos.

Fighting the fat

Fat is a concentrated source of energy: 1 g provides 9 calories. So, reducing fat aids weight loss. But fats slow carbohydrate absorption, helping to stave off hunger pangs and stabilize blood glucose levels. Indeed, many low GI foods can be high in fat. This means it's easy for a person with diabetes to eat too much fat.

Broadly, foods contain two types of fat:

- Unsaturated fat derives mainly from vegetables, nuts and seeds, and is usually liquid at room temperature. Olive, rapeseed, safflower and sunflower oils are unsaturated fats. There are two main subtypes: monounsaturated and polyunsaturated. Fish is especially high in a particularly beneficial type of polyunsaturated fat.
- Saturated fat comes mainly from animal sources – meat, full-fat dairy products, cakes, biscuits, pastries – and is generally solid at room temperature. The liver converts saturated fat into cholesterol.

Table 4 overleaf suggests some ways you could cut your consumption of saturated fat. The cooking method makes a big difference: grill, steam or oven-bake food instead of frying. If you must fry, use a small amount of olive oil at a low temperature. You could also try sautéing in a little water or tomato juice.

The trans fat danger

Many foods contain trans fats (also called trans fatty acids), which seem to markedly increase heart disease risk. Numerous foods, including cheese, cream, beef,

Table 4 Foods high in saturated fat and the low-fat alternative

	Avoid	*Low-fat alternative*
Snacks	Crisps/savoury snacks cooked in oil	Fresh or dried fruit, handful of nuts
Fats for cooking and spreading	Lard, dripping, ghee, cream and butter	Olive, sunflower, soya or rapeseed (blended vegetable) oils, margarines and spreads; store oils in a sealed container in a cool, dark place to prevent rancidity
Meat	Fatty products (sausages, burgers, pâté, salami, meat pies and pasties)	Lean cuts of meat and mince (check labels or ask the butcher); trim off fat Skinless chicken and turkey Vegetarian options (e.g. lentils, chickpeas and soya)
Fish	Deep fried (e.g. take-away) fish and chips	Oily fish such as salmon, mackerel and sardines
Sauces	Creamy or cheesy sauces	Tomato or vegetable-based sauces
Dairy	Full-fat varieties	Skimmed (or at least semi-skimmed) milk, reduced-fat cheddar and low-fat yoghurt Try grating cheese or using a strongly flavoured variety, which may mean you need to use less Edam, Camembert, Brie, reduced fat cheddar and cottage cheese contain less fat than many full-fat hard cheeses such as standard cheddar, Stilton, Parmesan and cream cheese

Source: Adapted from British Dietetic Association

lamb and mutton, naturally contain trans fats. But artificial trans fats – found in many processed foods – seem
to be especially hazardous.

Heating vegetable oils to fry foods creates trans
fats: one reason why it's better to steam, bake or grill.
Food production can convert vegetable oils into trans
fats ('hydrogenation'). Biscuits, pies and cakes as well
as some margarines and other spreads often contain
hydrogenated (or trans-unsaturated fats). Look for
foods labelled 'low in trans' or 'virtually trans-free', and
always check the label. Foods containing hydrogenated fats or hydrogenated vegetable oils almost always
include trans fatty acids.

Fish and omega-3 fatty acids

First Nation Arctic people seem to be less vulnerable
to several diseases, including diabetes, heart disease,
arthritis and asthma, than people in industrialized
countries. Yet their traditional diet consists almost
entirely of fish, seal and other animals that, in turn,
eat marine life. Fish oil is, however, rich in health-
boosting omega-3 polyunsaturated fatty acids (PUFAs,
also called n-3 fatty acids). Omega-3 PUFAs seem to
have several benefits, including:

- reducing inflammation;
- increasing levels of HDL;
- reducing triglyceride levels;
- lowering blood pressure;
- making blood less likely to clot;
- reducing the chance that an atherosclerotic plaque
  will burst.

So, eating oily fish reduces the risk of heart disease
and keeps your joints healthy. Omega-3 PUFAs are also

important for memory and mental performance, and, in experiments at least, protect eyes from damage from diabetes.

Omega-3 PUFAs – specifically docosahexaenoic acid (DHA) and eicosapentaenoic acid (EPA) – seem to be responsible for much of oily fish's benefit. We can make omega-3 fatty acids from another fat, alpha-lino-lenic acid, found in green leafy vegetables, nuts, seeds and their oils. But it's a slow process. So, boost levels by eating fish and seafood high in omega-3 PUFAs, such as tuna, salmon, herring, pilchard, mackerel, rainbow trout, dogfish, shrimp and crab. It's better to eat fresh fish. If you're eating canned fish, check the label to make sure processing has not depleted the omega-3 oils. It's also worth trying to check that the fish comes from sustainable stocks at <www.fishonline.org>.

If at first you don't like the taste, don't give up without trying a few recipes. There's plenty of choice on the internet and in cookery books. Poach, grill or bake rather than fry. And don't cover fish in bread-crumbs or batter, which can soak up fat. If you really can't stomach the taste of oily fish you could try a supplement. But speak to your doctor first. Omega-3 supplements (including cod liver oil) may increase blood sugar levels.

Oils, vitamin E and free radicals

A slice of apple exposed to the air soon turns brown. Tissue-damaging chemicals called free radicals cause the colour change. Free radicals are a by-product of the chemical reactions that keep us alive. Our immune system uses free radicals to help destroy invading bac-teria. But pollution, smoking, pesticides and sunlight can generate free radicals that attack healthy cells. Levels of free radicals rise in diabetes, which may contribute to some complications.

Several defences protect our cells from free radicals, such as vitamins, minerals and other antioxidants in our diets, including:

- vitamins A, C, E and selenium;
- lutein, found in, for example, green leafy vegetables such as spinach and kale;
- lycopene, the red pigment in tomatoes and some other fruits.

Oils are a natural source of vitamin E. Unfortunately, processing removes vitamin E from some oils. So, buy 'cold-pressed' vegetable oils from sources such as seeds, nuts and oily fish. Cold-pressed oils should last longer and help bolster your antioxidant intake.

Vegetables, fruit and fibre

Dietary fibre (roughage) is the part of plants that humans can't digest. There are two main types:

- Insoluble fibre remains largely intact as it moves through your digestive system, but eases defecation.
- Soluble fibre dissolves in water in the gut, forming a gel that soaks up fats. So a meal rich in soluble fibre means that you absorb less fat from a meal. Soluble fibre also releases sugar slowly.

A high-fibre diet slowly releases carbohydrate. This means you feel full for longer and you'll be less likely to snack between meals. A low-carbohydrate diet makes it easier to not eat enough wholemeal foods, fruit and vegetables. So, make sure you get enough:

- oats and oat bran
- fruit and vegetables
- nuts and seeds
- pulses – such as peas, soya, lentils and chickpeas
- wholemeal (wholegrain) breads and cereals (e.g. wheat, oats, rye, barley and corn).

Whole grains

Whole grains are an especially good source of fibre. Grains – the seeds of cereals, such as wheat, rye, barley, oats and rice – have three parts:

- Bran is the outer layer that is rich in fibre and packed with nutrients.
- The germ develops into a new plant and, again, is packed with nutrients. Wheat germ, for example, contains high levels of vitamin E, vitamin B_9 (folate/folic acid), zinc and magnesium, which may protect against diabetes.
- The central area (endosperm) is high in starch. The endosperm provides the energy the germ needs to develop into a new plant.

Food manufacturers refine grain by removing the bran and germ, leaving the white endosperm. So, whole grains contain up to 75 per cent more nutrients than refined cereals.

Regularly eating whole grains as part of a low-fat diet and a healthy lifestyle cuts the risk of heart disease and diabetes, and helps you control your weight and avoid hypos. So:

- Eat a bowl of porridge or muesli for breakfast every day.
- Eat stoneground wholewheat bread.

- Use brown or basmati rice instead of white rice.
- Use wholewheat pasta instead of refined white pasta.
- Include whole grains, such as barley, in soups and stews.
- Use bulgur wheat in casseroles and stir-fries.
- Substitute half the refined white flour in pancakes, buns and other flour-based recipes with wholewheat or oat flour.
- Use rolled oats or crushed unsweetened wholegrain cereal instead of bread to coat chicken, fish and so on.
- Use wholegrain flour or oatmeal when baking.

Five portions of fruit and vegetables

Make sure you eat at least five portions of fruit and vegetables a day. A portion weighs about 80 g – that's about the same as:

- one medium-sized fruit (banana, apple, pear, orange)
- one slice of a large fruit (melon, pineapple, mango)
- two smaller fruits (plums, satsumas, apricots, peaches)
- a dessert bowl full of salad
- three heaped tablespoons of pulses (chickpeas, lentils, beans)
- two to three tablespoons (a handful) of grapes or berries
- one tablespoon of dried fruit
- one glass (150 ml) of unsweetened fruit or vegetable juice or smoothie. Two or more glasses still only count as one portion.

To get the most benefit:

- Eat fruit and vegetables as raw as possible. Cook vegetables using the minimum of unsalted (or lightly salted) water; lightly steam or stir-fry.
- Scrub rather than peel: the skin can contain valuable nutrients.
- Freeze any fruit and vegetables you can't eat straight away.
- When buying tinned fruit, choose those in 100 per cent fruit juice rather than syrup.
- Don't buy vegetables that come with sauces that contain added salt, sugar or fats.
- Don't soak prepared fruit or vegetables, which may dissolve some vitamins and minerals.

Try the following to boost your intake:

- Drink smoothies. Two whole portions of fruit in a homemade smoothie counts as two of your five portions. Some commercial smoothies contain extra sugar, honey, yoghurt or milk that can increase the calorie, fat and sugar content. Always check the label.
- Snack on oranges, bananas, grapes, dried apricots, peaches, pineapple slices, baby carrots or celery sticks.
- Add crushed fresh pineapple to coleslaw and mandarin oranges or grapes to a salad.
- Try baked apples, pears or a fruit salad for dessert.
- Try to eat a green salad every day as a main meal or side salad, or at work.
- Plan some meals around vegetables, such as stir-fries, curries and soups.
- Add chopped vegetables to a pasta sauce or lasagne.

- Use cooked and pureed vegetables such as potatoes to thicken soup, stew or gravy.
- Barbecue vegetable kebabs.

However, fruits are packed with a sugar called fructose. So, eating large amounts of fruit in a short time can drive your blood glucose levels up.

Seeds, nuts and legumes

Seeds, nuts and legumes are an excellent source of fibre and nutrients. Sunflower, sesame, hemp, flax and pumpkin seeds can be:

- eaten as snacks;
- sprinkled on to porridge and other breakfast cereals, as well as over salads;
- added to vegetable or meat dishes and soups;
- used in baking.

For more flavour, lightly roast the seeds after coating with soy sauce. Cracked linseed and pumpkin seeds are highly nutritious and can help alleviate constipation. However, seeds are relatively high in calories, so eat in moderation if you are trying to lose weight. Eat a handful a day of almonds, cashews, walnuts, Brazils and pecans as snacks, with cereal and in baking.

Legumes are a cheap source of protein, have relatively little effect on blood glucose levels, are high in fibre and help control levels of fats in the blood. Legumes include:

- baked beans
- kidney beans
- chickpeas
- red and green lentils

- mung beans
- butter beans
- black beans
- split peas
- haricot beans.

Use beans in stews, soups, salads and casseroles and eat one to three portions of legumes daily. One portion is three heaped tablespoons. The soya bean is rich in PUFAs and low in saturated fat. One portion of soya beans counts towards your five portions of fruits and vegetables a day, is high in fibre and contains all the essential amino acids.

Salt

High levels of salt (sodium chloride) in your blood can damage your cells. So, your body retains fluid to dilute the salt, which drives blood pressure up. This means that a high intake of salt makes hypertension more likely, which can lead to strokes and heart disease.

You can tell that some snacks are salty. But many processed and pre-packaged foods contain hidden salt added as a preservative and flavour enhancer. Indeed, manufacturers may add surprisingly large amounts of salt to some soups, bread, biscuits and breakfast cereals and even fresh chicken and turkey.

To cut your salt intake:

- Avoid foods that are high in salt, such as smoked meat and fish.
- Use as little salt as you can during baking and cooking.
- Banish the salt cellar from the table.

- Ask restaurants and take-aways for no salt.
- Use low-salt ketchup, pickled items, mustard, yeast extract and stock cubes.

Food may taste bland when you first reduce your salt use, but you'll soon adjust. In a few weeks you will probably wonder why you preferred your foods so salty.

8

Using supplements safely

In theory, you shouldn't need vitamin and mineral supplements if you eat a healthy balanced diet. Nevertheless, some people use supplements as insurance policies, or to treat or prevent a health problem. They may want to try herbs to keep their glucose levels down, tackle a complication or help another disease. However, people with diabetes need to be careful. Manganese and vanadium, for example, augment insulin's action and could trigger a hypo. So, check with your diabetes team. Indeed, everyone taking a medicine for any disease *must* speak to a doctor or nurse before taking supplements.

Alpha-lipoic acid

Cells produce a chemical called alpha-lipoic acid to help generate energy. In addition, alpha-lipoic acid, also known as thioctic acid, seems to:

- mop up free radicals;
- help recycle other antioxidants, including vitamins C and E;
- improve blood flow to nerves and enhance nerve conduction;
- prevent destruction of beta cells;
- enhance glucose uptake by cells;
- slow the development of diabetic complications, including neuropathy.

Doctors in some countries can prescribe alpha-lipoic acid to treat diabetic neuropathy. In the UK, you can buy alpha-lipoic acid from health food shops. High doses can cause headache, rash and stomach upsets and trigger hypoglycaemia.

Chromium

Chromium boosts the action of insulin and helps the body use protein, fat and carbohydrate effectively. In some animal experiments, chromium supplements prevented the development of diabetes. In places in the world where the soil contains little chromium, supplementation reverses some cases of diabetes. Whole grains, meat, egg yolk, mushrooms and meat are rich in chromium.

Magnesium

Several studies suggest that taking about 400 mg of magnesium a day seems to reduce diabetes risk by a third compared with an intake of about 250 mg a day. Boost your consumption by eating more whole grains, legumes, nuts and beans.

Vanadium

Large doses (100–125 mg/day) of vanadium improve cells' sensitivity to insulin in humans. But at these doses, vanadium tends to cause side effects such as abdominal discomfort, diarrhoea, nausea, flatulence, loss of energy and even a green tongue. Future studies need to investigate whether vanadium is safe and effective in preventing diabetes.

Vitamin B$_{12}$ (cyanocobalamin)

Vitamin B$_{12}$ is essential:

- for formation of red blood cells;
- to produce DNA, which carries your genetic code;
- to make sure your nerves work properly;
- and to help the body use fat and protein effectively.

Animal products – such as oily fish, seafood, meat, eggs, milk and poultry – contain vitamin B$_{12}$. Some breakfast cereals are fortified with vitamin B$_{12}$.

Vitamin B$_{12}$ supplements may improve:

- diabetic neuropathy, reducing pain and paraesthesia (sensations such as tingling, burning, pricking and pins and needles);
- autonomic symptoms caused by nerve damage, which include constipation, diarrhoea, impotence, dry skin and poor awareness of hypoglycaemia.

Further studies are needed. Nevertheless, if you've developed neuropathy speak to your diabetes team about taking vitamin B$_{12}$.

Vitamin C (ascorbic acid)

Vitamin C is one of the body's most important defences against free radicals, which rise in diabetes and may contribute to some complications. Vitamin C may also reduce formation by the body of a sugar called sorbitol that's linked to retinopathy, neuropathy and kidney damage.

In one study, almost three in five people with diabetes showed low levels of vitamin C in their blood. Other studies suggest that, on average, people with diabetes have vitamin C levels that are around a third lower than healthy people. While vitamin C supplements don't markedly change blood glucose levels, sorbitol levels decline and the capillaries may become less fragile. Raw cabbage, carrots, lettuce, onions, celery, tomatoes, oranges, lemons, limes, grapefruits and all other citrus fruits are good sources of vitamin C.

Herbal supplements

Metformin, a widely used diabetes drug, is a chemical modification of substances in goat's rue, also called French lilac (*Galega officinalis*), which medieval healers used to relieve the urinary problems that accompany diabetes. Fenugreek (*Trigonella foenum-graecum*) can lower blood glucose levels to a similar extent as insulin.

So, some herbs could trigger a hypo. But if you're using diet alone to treat T2DM or you are still in prediabetes, some of these herbal supplements may help control blood glucose levels. However, everyone taking a medicine for diabetes or any other disease *must* speak to a doctor or diabetes nurse before taking a herbal treatment – even one bought from a health shop. Indeed, it's best to be treated by a qualified medical herbalist. Make sure that your herbalist knows you have diabetes and any other conditions. Contact the National Institute of Medical Herbalists (<www.nimh.org.uk>).

Bitter melon

Bitter melon (*Momordica charantia*), also called bitter gourd or balsam pear, is a traditional treatment for diabetes across Asia, South America, India and East Africa. Numerous studies performed since the 1950s show that bitter melon lowers blood glucose levels – in some investigations as much as certain drugs for diabetes.

Bitter melon helps cells use glucose more efficiently, reduces insulin resistance and lowers glucose levels. In one study of people with T2DM, bitter melon reduced glucose levels by, on average, about one-fifth. Around nine in ten patients with T2DM benefited. Gastrointestinal upset is a possible side effect and children occasionally developed diabetic coma after drinking bitter melon tea. Further investigations are needed to fully define the benefits.

Evening primrose oil

Oil from the seeds of the evening primrose (*Oenothera biennis*) are high in omega-3 and omega-6 PUFAs, which are essential for normal nerve activity. Some studies involving people with diabetic neuropathy found that evening primrose oil might improve nerve function and alleviate symptoms. More studies are needed before doctors can routinely suggest the treatment. But if you want to try evening primrose oil, speak to your doctor or diabetes nurse.

Fenugreek

Fenugreek seems to stimulate insulin secretion and reduce insulin resistance. Indeed, in some studies, fenugreek lowered blood glucose to a similar extent as insulin. Fenugreek seeds are high in fibre and slow glucose absorption after a meal. In addition, fenugreek reduces levels of triglycerides, cholesterol and LDL-cholesterol.

Ginseng

Ginseng (*Panax ginseng* and *Panax quinquefolius*) seems to:

- boost the immune system;
- reduce inflammation and mop up free radicals;
- improve the conversion of glucose into energy;
- protect insulin-producing beta cells from destruction;
- almost halve the peak in glucose after eating;
- normalize insulin levels;
- reduce cholesterol levels and weight.

So, ginseng seems to reduce the risk of cardiovascular disease and infections. In studies of people with T2DM, ginseng, among other benefits:

- blunted the surge in glucose levels after a meal;
- reduced HbA_{1c};
- reduced fasting glucose levels;
- increased levels of physical activity.

Prickly pear

Several small studies suggest that the prickly pear (*Opuntia humifusa*) may lower blood glucose levels. In an experiment using diabetic rats, an extract of prickly pear reduced levels of blood glucose, triglycerides, cholesterol and LDL-cholesterol, while boosting HDL-cholesterol. If this high-fibre fruit is not available in your local greengrocer, you could drink prickly pear as a powder or juice from a health food shop.

Benefits and limitations

As these examples illustrate, numerous herbs and
supplements may improve diabetes, according
to scientific studies, medical traditions or both.
Nevertheless, few complementary therapies undergo
the same rigorous scrutiny as modern medicines.
This isn't surprising: clinical studies are expensive
and drug companies fund most trials. No evidence
of effectiveness isn't necessarily the same as evidence
of no effect. Nevertheless, stop using the supplement
if you fail to see any benefits after three months or
suffer side effects. Before starting a course of herbal
supplements, speak to your GP or diabetes care team.
Ideally, see a medical herbalist – and let him or her
know you have diabetes.

Summing up

This brief book explains how a healthy lifestyle and
diet will help you control your blood glucose levels
and protect against diabetic complications. As you
change your lifestyle, you'll need to keep an eye
on your blood glucose level – assuming you're not
making the changes to tackle prediabetes or treat early
T2DM.

A healthy, balanced diet should help you lose any
excess weight and stay at a healthy body BMI. If you
can eat healthily, have portions of the recommended
size and become more active, you will lose weight. So,
you may need to adjust your medications to control
your blood sugar levels. It's important that you speak
to your doctor or diabetes care team. But even if the
drugs remain the same, a healthy lifestyle and balanced

diet will help you reduce the risk that you'll develop the serious complications often linked to diabetes. You really are what you eat.